# Walks With Cancer

## In Steps With Hope

Mirella Coacci van der Zyl

**Walks With Cancer – In Steps With Hope**



Author's Note: All stories in this book are told through the author's eyes, except where noted otherwise. The author has permission to tell the stories of all participants in her book.

Ordering Information:
Books may be ordered directly through Amazon or by contacting the author, mirellavanderzyl@gmail.com
Discounts are available for volume orders.

ISBN 9798568394273

Note: this book was edited and compiled with the assistance of the team at Cavern of Dreams Publishing in Brantford, Ontario, Canada

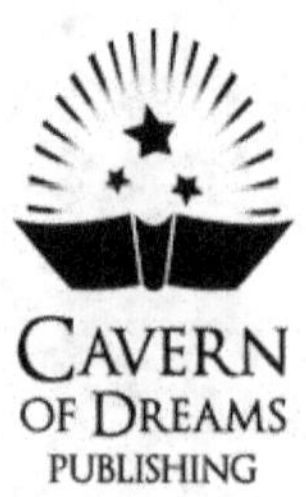

CAVERN
OF DREAMS
PUBLISHING

*Other Titles*

*by*

*Mirella Coacci van der Zyl*

On Call for God

I Heard the Rumbling of Planes

Silva's Journey

Nona's Chair

Bullied

*Dedicated to the memory of my dear sister,*

*Paola Coacci-Cushnie,*

*who lost her battle with cancer.*

*"In the midst of all circumstances, God's grace, peace, and joy are there."*

*-Billy Graham*

# *Introduction*

There are many books and articles written about surviving disaster, violence, or illness. I survived cancer twice in my life: how can I deal with such a miracle? It is a miracle, in every sense to me, because I am alive and well, and enjoying my golden years. I attribute this miracle to God, my Healer.

I decided to share some of my experiences with my readers. My words may bring comfort to some individuals; others may see hope for their future. Still, others might discard my words as useless. As I share my journey with cancer, much of my focus will also be on my personal journey with the Lord Jesus Christ. Christ has been a large part of my life, and I felt His presence most prominently when I was going through my illness.

Another person who supported me significantly during this trying time was my beloved mother, who came to reside with me when I first learned about my illness. She was a nurse before she stayed home with her children and helped my father in his Ministry of our Baptist Church in Italy. She knew how to make me comfortable and feel well cared for.

My life was changing. For a time, I thought it was over; I didn't want to talk to anyone, not even my mother. I closed up and shut everybody out. Only two or three people knew about my condition, and I made sure to keep it that way for a while. Why? There was a sense of confusion within me. I thought I had done something wrong in my life, and this cancer was the punishment for my transgressions. So, I kept quiet and lived with it—by myself. However, eventually, my attitude changed. As you read on, I will make light of it.

I ask you to journey with me through my experiences with cancer, plus the experiences of others who wished to share their story with me. I will end with my husband's story, as he not only assisted me through my cancer scares but had his own.

# Part One

# My Story

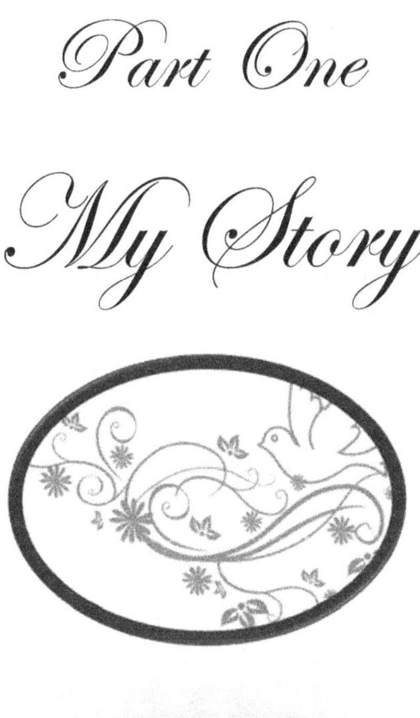

# *My Concept of Cancer*

From readings, conversations with other people, and my doctor's comments, I gathered information about this mysterious disease. Cancer is a group of malignant cells that grow on an organ and spread to different body areas—metastasis.

In some cases, cancer can be so aggressive that chemotherapy, radiation, surgery, and medications cannot stop the disease from spreading. In a short time, the body cannot fight it any longer, and complications, including death, may occur. Such was the case for my younger sister, who lost her cancer battle at too young an age.

In fortunate cases, cancer doesn't spread. Surgery removes the affected part, and with medication, the patient may be free for many years. Such was the way it was for me the first time.

My husband also developed cancer—a benign mass in the prostate, which continues to sit there. His surgeon checks it once every six months, but there is no growth or spreading, and my husband feels fine.

Why are there so many different aspects of cancer? Billy Graham said, *"In the midst of all circumstances, God's grace, peace, and joy are there."*—a harsh statement for many people to accept. Several people, who suffer because of cancer, say, "Where is God in all of this?"

Even though I was a pastor, ministering to those in hospitals, I should have been more positive. Faced with my own illness, though, I had no words to reassure them God was in the midst of their suffering. I had no arguments to help them cope, to give them the courage to fight one day at a time. How could I say these things if, at times, I struggled to believe them myself? We are all human when these sorts of things enter our lives.

However, as I moved through my days with cancer, I slowly came to believe Billy Graham's words and hold them precious. There was a level of realism some days when I was strong enough to cope with my illness.

# The Beginning

My journey started with a simple visit to my doctor. He noticed an unusual lump in my breast; however, he dismissed it as a cyst. After we moved to a different city, the new doctor I saw wasn't impressed with my X-Ray. It showed calcium on my breast, and she sent me to an oncologist who discovered that the lump was malignant.

Leaving the oncologist's office, after he told me I needed a mastectomy, I was numb. I hardly noticed that my friend, Libby, had taken me home. She was very comforting and supportive of me, but I was so distraught I barely responded to her attempts.

However, my beloved friend persisted, and Libby gave me the courage and the determination to proceed with the mastectomy the doctor suggested. It saved my life because, now, after twenty-seven years, I have had no recurrence of breast cancer.

I told the news to Ernest, my husband, my daughter, who lived with us, and my mother, who lived in North Carolina. I didn't want to talk to anybody else about my situation. I kept the apprehension for the up-coming surgery within myself. And most of all, I worried about how my body would look after the operation. I had always been vigilant with the care of my body—my health—and I couldn't explain this malignancy—how it was going to change my body.

I began to blame myself for my misfortune. What had I done wrong? Negative thoughts continued to plague me. I refused to talk about my feelings to anybody because deep within me were moods of guilt, shame, and resentment. How would my friends and family feel towards me now, once they found out I had cancer? Once again, my faith in God was shaken, and I wondered how I was to minister to others.

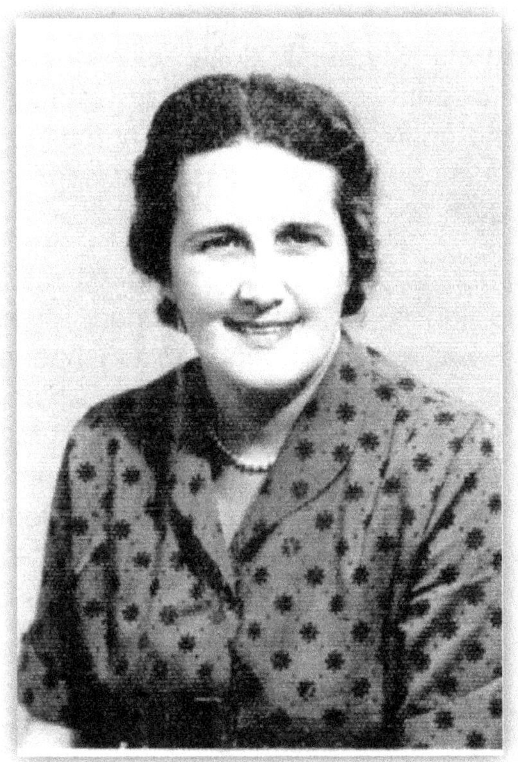

*(My Mother)*

And then, my dear mother came to me. She decided to stay until I was able to return to work. She gave me her undivided attention and care and tried to talk to me about hope for the future. There were tears in her eyes when she spoke.

Ernest was working in another town during my illness and wasn't able to be with me all the time; however, he compensated on the weekends by helping out around the house. My daughter, who was only 19 at the time, never told me how she felt about me having breast cancer, and I allowed her to have her privacy.

On the morning of my surgery, my mother and Libby accompanied me. My family doctor was there as well and reassured me that she would stay with the surgeon throughout the entire procedure. The nurses couldn't have been more caring and considerate towards me, and I healed quickly in the hospital.

My friend and my daughter picked me up when it was time to leave the hospital. Once I was home, I discovered I was much stronger than I had been giving myself credit for. I walked into my home, which my mother had made tidy and comfortable, and sank into a freshly made bed, thankful for the softness—compared to the hospital beds—as well as the quietness. I slept for a long time, and when I awoke, I surprised my mother and my daughter by getting up and dressing without assistance.

# A Sense of Relief

Well, it was over! Or was it? There came a time of waiting, long, nerve-wracking waiting. During the surgery, the surgeons took nodes from under my arm to investigate if cancer had spread there. On my next visit to Juravinski hospital, the doctor told me there was no cancer detected. I needed to take *Tamoxifen*, though, a medication that attaches to the hormone receptors in the cancer cell, blocking estrogen from attaching to the receptors, slowing or stopping the tumour's growth by preventing the cancer cells from getting the hormones they need to grow. I was to take this medication for five years and return for a check-up every six months. I was free of cancer; my heart cried jubilantly! A sense of relief overwhelmed me, and I could talk to my family freely now that it was all over. I felt whole again, healthy and alive—I was me once more!

I still didn't talk much about the ordeal—Libby being the only person outside my family to whom I had confided. But, somehow, the news spread around my church, and a few visitors came to see me. I believe this happened because one of the ministers was seeing other patients in the hospital, saw my name, and visited me.

My husband worked hard on weekends when he was home to make the house more comfortable for us. I sincerely appreciated how he tried to understand what I was going through. He reassured me immensely that he did not find me unattractive now, but he had more love and tenderness for me. He helped me to recover as much as he knew how.

I spent lovely weekends with my family, and it was a bonus having my mom and my daughter preparing delightful meals. My mom was a fabulous cook and spoiled all of us quite a bit. Not to toot my horn here, but I believe I have taken after Mom and my paternal grandmother because I'm a good cook too. My husband always refers to me as *"my Bella cuoce,"* meaning, "my beautiful cook."

My mom and I went shopping several times, and she was amazed I could drive my car with such ease. I could move my arm without pain, and this reassured me that I was on the mend. I decided to take even better care of myself by doing something special for me, so I went to the hairdresser, bought a nice outfit, and started to enjoy my life again.

Four weeks after I had the mastectomy, the doctor cleared me to return to work, and I surprised my fellow chaplains in the hospital for being strong enough to work again. I loved being a chaplain, and now I could add my own experience in knowing how it was to go through cancer surgery—the waiting for results, the recovery, etc.

However, I met several patients who hadn't been as fortunate with the outcome as I had been. Their cancer was still active and painful, rendering them hopeless. I tried my best to comfort and love the patients because I knew first-hand what was happening to them. Some of them remained angry with God, though, and refused prayer.

# Coping with my New Life

*"But I will restore you to health and heal your wounds,"*
*declares the Lord. -Jeremiah 30:17*

**It happened with a burst** of light! I found this verse in the bible. One day I was feeling depressed thinking about the possibility of getting cancer again. It disheartened me, as well, about the people I had ministered to, especially those who had no hope. My faith was becoming lukewarm, and I was beginning to question why God would allow so much suffering in the world. Some people got better, while others suffered terribly and died early. Why was it so?

One day, with this attitude, I was checking my bible, in which I had marked some notable passages, when I came upon Jeremiah 30:17. I read it several times, stunned by its promise. Could it be that God indeed restored sick people to health? Why some he did, and some he didn't? Or so it appeared to me.

I clung to the cross and rested there, asking for advice. It came to me in the form of a magazine article. It depends a lot on our genes, how we form physically when conceived, and how we grow later. Countless issues may improve our health, while others may destroy our good genes and bring us closer to death. It all boils down to how we are made. Smoking, drinking, living a sedentary life, and our diet—yes, these are all factors that may worsen our health situations. We all know this. But sometimes, even the healthiest individuals are struck down with an illness.

After much thought, I returned to the bible passage and have kept it precious for use in my life and my ministry.

# Still Learning and Growing

Slowly, my attitude changed towards myself and my life. I still didn't talk to my friends and family about what I had gone through. I didn't want to share with anybody, not even my mom, that I felt pain in that part of my body. I did exercise a bit, and then when spring came, I went for short walks in the neighbourhood. There were times when, as I was walking and enjoying the trees becoming green again, I felt alive, pulsating with a will to live, to go on with my work, to create something. I knew my family and friends cared for me, but they left me alone, not wanting to intrude.

The words of the prophet Jeremiah kept coming to my mind. They vibrated with a sure promise for me because I was healing well and feeling healthier. My spirit began lifting to an expectant level, where I felt my health slowly restored. I began to feel I could leave behind surgery and sickness experiences and enjoy a wholesome life again. My death time was not approaching me yet, and God's promise kept me praying for future years without cancer.

My work at the hospital became even more significant to me. I discovered myself finding more words of assurance and more faith to share with the residents—especially those in palliative care. My visits with them became more intense, and, at times, even without mentioning God or His promises, my words and my presence brought some comfort and support to the sick person. Prayer became vital in our visit and, after the ill person relaxed, telling me how they felt God was near and listening. They felt a prayer was beneficial, no matter if they believed in God or not.

My compassion for the sick people became more profound, and my love for people, no matter their condition, swelled within me. I didn't give much thought to my personal battle with cancer. It appeared that my body was healing well, and I was gaining strength. I couldn't be indifferent to other cancer patients. Some wanted to die soon, while others thought that was God's will for them— that they should suffer.

"In this life, we have to suffer because that's what God wants for us." I heard these words often spoken through tears of sorrow and pain. Even if I disagreed with them, I would respect the feelings of that person. Jeremiah's words were always present in these conversations. I would convey to these people that even though it didn't look like the disease would be cured in this life, there was a promise and hope of perfect health, no suffering, and no tears the moment we would be with the Lord. With Him, there would be perfect peace in the place where He would take us. Several prophets proclaimed we would be in a place where the days of our sorrow and suffering will be no more, which is something I believe in firmly and passed on to others.

*"I can do everything through Him who gives me strength." -*
*Philippians 4:13*

The above verse, which I learned in my early years of Sunday School, became my motto. I shared it with many people in my care and with my friends. The patients would smile and repeat it, and I could see it made them feel content and relaxed.

Eventually, I found a place where they could make prostheses for me, and I began to feel more normal when I dressed and undressed. I avoided touching my scar or looking at it any more than I had to. It only reminded me of a dark stage of my life, but now I was looking at a bright sky, building a stronger hope with each passing day.

# *Hope*

Hope became the key word in my life, and I shared it repeatedly. There were still people whose attitude towards the disease would allow it to take hold of them, taking them into a dark tunnel of hopelessness as they considered the effects of the disease and the therapies facing them. Many of these same people also detached themselves from family and friends.

I once heard someone state that life was greater than cancer. This statement is so true, and I have had the opportunity to witness this in my own life. Not too long ago, I heard a lady say, "I'm not well today. We need to suffer. That is good; God wants us to suffer in this life." It stunned me to hear this contrasting statement, especially on a beautiful, sunny day of summer.

The God I know and worship is a God of infinite love. He does not want us to suffer because He gave us a life to enjoy many good experiences. God provides us with the strength and ability to cope with our sicknesses, with our losses, and with financial difficulties. One way or the other, I have witnessed how He helped me cope and advance through all those experiences. I came out of them much sturdier and with more trust in my providing Lord.

As my experience with cancer got further in the past, I noticed how my health was improving. Hope for my future to be cancer-free surged in me like a brilliant light, and I looked at my life with new hope and joy.

Family and friends watched me, and I received countless beautiful cards with expressions of support. I treasured them, and I still keep them until today.

My greatest wish is to share my hopes of a cancer-free future with all those whose view of life is so negative. I believe God is one of love and care, who does not abandon His children in despair but gathers them in His arms if they go to Him and stay with Him.

I am aware that some people may not have my faith, but I would like to say that God may not heal everyone who contracts the disease, but He gives the ability to cope with the disease's progress in the end.

# Part Two:

# The Second Time Around

# *And then, it happened again.*

One day, after I had retired and enjoyed life at home, I touched my neck, and it felt quite swollen. Fear gripped my stomach. *Here we go again*, I thought. This time I felt as though a death sentence was handed to me. I thought, this time, my life was over. Usually, I felt very well, but I knew something was wrong again in my body, and so, the process began all over again. I started another round of doctors' visits and blood tests. I was filled with dread, waiting for results.

Once again, my beloved friend, Libby, stood by my side, but my dear mother had since passed away. I had been cancer-free for seventeen years, living a serene, bright life, happy with my work, followed by retirement, and writing my books.

This time, the oncologist suggested a biopsy of my thyroid; he suspected that was causing my trouble. I had to go through more tests, and then the week of my biopsy came around.

# *Beloved, in loving arms*

**Ernest has been with me** throughout this journey, and he took me to the hospital early in the morning for my biopsy. I was extremely nervous because this meant something serious was going on. I was given a bed, and my husband sat by my side. I waited for what felt like a dreadfully long time, my apprehension increasing with each passing hour. When I couldn't stand the anxiety any longer, I thought of my Lord on the cross and how He must have felt hanging there in agony.

Suddenly I felt lifted in a warm, tender embrace, and I felt comforted. It was a peaceful and calming feeling that lasted the rest of the morning. It dawned on me that I knew some of my church friends were praying for me that day, and this gave me a sense of calm and relaxation, knowing how much I was loved.

By the time the nurses wheeled me into a room full of machinery and people in green scrubs, I felt calmer. However, my heart monitor didn't relay my calmness; it showed a rapid heartbeat. The nurses gave me medication to help my heart rate slow down, and soon it became stable again. From that point, everything moved along quickly, and soon enough, we were on our way home.

The biopsy was quite an ordeal for me, but now the worst part had begun—waiting for my results. I had to wait a week, and with Libby, I headed to the hospital to find out my results. I wasn't surprised in the slightest with the doctor's verdict. I had follicular lymphoma in my chest, and it was attacking my thyroid. A few sessions of chemo would clear it out, the doctor had assured me.

"I am not much use to you now," my friend had cried to me. I was numb and didn't want to dwell on that word—lymphoma, mostly because my dear sister, Paola, had passed away from that horrid disease.

I had always thought of it as a *light cancer*, but I had to have more tests to see if cancer had invaded my bones. Once again, I was fortunate that it hadn't spread to other parts of my body. Now I was thinking about having chemo and was terrified. Why me?

# Fear of the Unknown Sickness

Many thoughts occurred to me about having chemo. What if I got dreadfully sick and couldn't keep up with my tasks at home, in the church, and other volunteer activities? What if I lost my hair that I cherished so? What if I lost the sharpness of my mind?

At the church, we had times of special prayer for those who needed it. It took a lot of courage to join my prayer partners and confess that I was afraid of the coming chemo. The partners prayed with me, and I felt my courage growing inside, and I began trusting more in the Lord's help. I finally believed I was ready to face this next test.

When I heard stories about cancer, surgery, chemo, radiation, I shuddered and quieted myself away for a while. But then I would revive and tell myself every story is different. My first encounter with cancer was unique to me because it was my story. We are all individuals, and the outcome of treatments, medications, and recovery will not be the same for everyone.

The next round of chemo sessions began. Ernest, my beloved, ever-faithful husband, drove me to the clinic and stayed with me through the hours. I watched the drip, falling slowly into my arm, and wondered if it would heal me or damage my body more. I was determined to take the hours as they came—at the clinic and home—without thinking fearful thoughts. It will be what it will be was my attitude.

I was amazed when the only symptom I felt from the chemo was hunger. I was ravenous, and the nurses very kindly gave me something to eat. I started to bring in my crochet work, and with my husband sitting next to me, I waited patiently for the drips to end. When I got home, I usually prepared a good supper and relaxed in front of the TV. For that week, this ordeal was over.

Over the next few days, I expected symptoms and reactions to develop, but I felt only tiredness. I went on with my household tasks and decided to start a journal about my thoughts and reactions.

In the beginning, I went for treatments once a week for three weeks in a row. Treatments would stop for a few weeks, and then another session would begin. This scenario went on for two years, intravenously, for several hours at the clinic. Thank goodness Ernest was retired and was able to be with me. He continued to be my rock.

Time went by quickly between my chemo sessions. Slowly, my fears and apprehension diminished: I wasn't losing my hair, only a few strands left on my pillow; however, I couldn't go to the hairdresser as I would have liked because when one is on chemo, they have to be careful due to a compromised immune system. Chemo not only destroys the bad cells, but it can also kill good cells. I guess I was lucky in some ways—wasn't losing weight or my appetite, and I continued to take good care of my body and paid attention to how I looked and dressed. Plus, I made sure I smiled often.

After a few months, I noticed that my chemo and cancer experience was simple, not as disastrous as other people revealed. My doctors told me that my type of lymphoma was easily curable. I realized how lucky I was, even if the chemo had left me exhausted most of the time.

Soon, two years had passed with numerous sessions of chemo. Finally, the day came when my doctor announced that it would be my final chemo treatment. I would only have to return every three months for a check-up. The clinic staff had been most gracious and helpful, and they were happy to see me go home. This ordeal was finally over. However, now I was wary and couldn't help but wonder—what was next on the horizon for me?

# *What is your purpose for me, O Lord?*

Now, I am home, resuming my everyday life, and perhaps I am even more attentive and caring for my family because I know I may leave them. I am thinking more about my demise and how I may pass away before others in my family. I imagined how each member of my family would take my passing. It brought tears to my eyes, and I decided not to dwell on those thoughts anymore. This time, though, I kept in mind that cancer might strike again in my life—I may never be free of it. I felt my life should be more useful and caring for others.

I started looking over my papers, collected during my years of studies. I realized I received an extensive education, more than average. I was retired, but could I not use my knowledge in some way still? My thoughts reached for the Lord, searching for guidance, asking Him what was still ahead in my life?

*"Weeping may endure for a night, but joy comes in the morning," King James- Psalm 30:5*

As I searched my bible, this verse caught my eye. I felt like I had endured a dismal night filled with discomfort and anxiety, but at the end of the darkness, there stretched a plane of joy for me. Was this the joy promised to me?

As I continued my search through my accumulated papers, the realization that there was a lot of material depicting my work over the past years brought me to a decision: I would write what transpired based on my writings. There were anecdotes, meditations, revelations, thoughts, and prayers.

Thus, my second career as a writer began. Since my school years, I have always kept diaries and wrote stories, sermons, essays, etc. Some of them were good enough that my teachers would read them aloud to the class. In grade five, I won a regional prize in a competition about rice cultivation in Italy. I learned a lot in preparing that composition.

Once I decided to become a writer—possibly a published writer—it was easy to start, using some of my papers' ideas. Honestly, it gave me great pleasure. Here was the joy the Psalmist mentioned. Despite the dark periods in my life, now there was pure happiness approaching on the horizon. It excited me to express my thoughts and feelings, sharing my hope for days to come with my readers.

I know I'm not the best writer, partly because my mother tongue is not English, but I have spent many years learning and honing it. I began writing in English around the time I was twelve. Most of these stories are lost now, but at the time, my teachers would read them to the class and say this is the way to write stories. Most of my tales were about my life and my pets.

I thought, possibly, I wouldn't be good enough to be published, but I would try anyway because it gave me great joy to gather my thoughts, ponder my stories, and put them on paper. I was proud of my accomplishments every time I completed a page. I don't know the outcome of this new enterprise, and at the moment, I think it is to glorify my Lord in my writing and make Him known to my future readers.

My prayer now is, "My Lord, if this is Your purpose for the rest of my life, You may bring it to success, and that it may bring the knowledge of You and Your love to many places."

# The thread of hope continues

The hope for a healthy future continues in my life. For now, I have days where I feel well and creative and other days where I don't. Despite the down days, I am pushing forward, taking the days as they come.

Visits to my oncologist have shown promising results. He feels I am one of his most successful patients, and he decided he didn't need to see me as often.

Slowly, my anxiety for future bouts of cancer is diminishing. Hope is a beautiful channel of light. It is like a thread—a golden thread in our hands. We roll it around between our fingers and keep it precious. Hope is like a small bird that knows it can fly but lingers on the tree branch, staying there for a while.

My hope is in Jesus Christ. I trust in Him that He will continue to walk with me in my life, whatever turn I take. I may be in remission of my cancer, or not, but the hope of better days in health and strength stays with me. Jesus Christ guides me by the hand and helps me cope with whatever discomfort I have; I firmly believe He can do it. My hope is that you will be able to feel the same as I do.

How is my life now?—after more than seven years since my last bout of cancer? It is serene and calm. Health wise, I endure the times of un-wellness as the years pass. I don't look my age, nor do I feel it, but pains and difficulties in completing my tasks come sometimes. Arthritis has slowed me down and makes me tired. It comes to everyone with the advancement of age, and there is little we can do except to take good care of ourselves. However, the doctor says I am healthy and hardly look my age, so I am to keep it up whatever I am doing. He even went as far as to ask me what my secret was!

At the moment, I feel free from cancer, but I try not to take this miracle for granted. I am in remission, but I realize it may raise its head again.

These days, I keep myself busy with housekeeping, which I love, and I also spend time writing. There are several books I would still like to write before my end. In all of them, I would like to keep the spirit of hope in Christ alive. Mostly these days, though, I take care of my dear Ernest, who isn't well. We married "in sickness and in health," which I respect and keep present those vows in my life. When writing this account, we are spending a quiet, pleasant life together in a retirement community, still living independently in our own accommodation. The home has numerous programs we can participate in, and I do my best to get Ernest involved.

Hope is leading me ahead with a good outlook of the future because it's in the hands of my Lord.

*"Then sing my soul, my Saviour God to Thee, How great Thou art, how great Thou art."*

# Part Three:

# Different voices~~

# Different experiences

I have shared my story with you, but I know many more stories of people who went through what I went through. Several didn't win their battle, and others are still struggling with the disease and therapy.

I thought to interview some of these individuals and see what we can learn from them—what their courage and hope might show us.

# Paola's Story

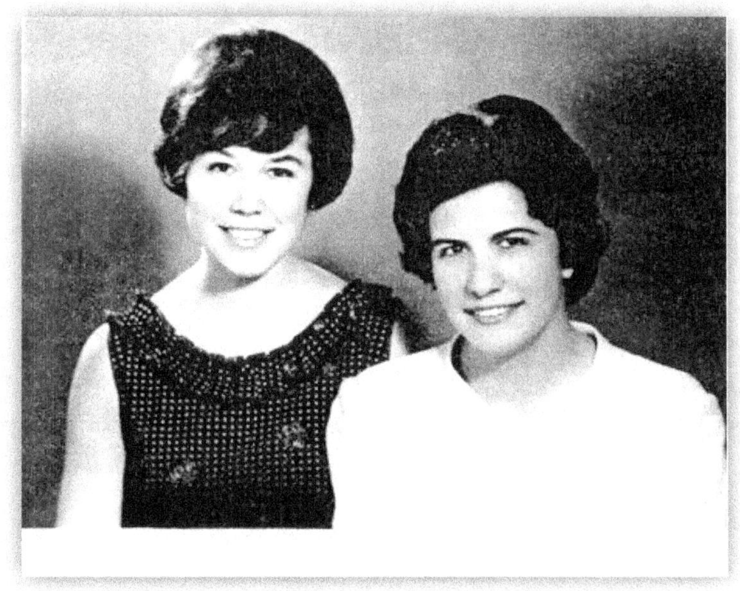

*(Paola and me)*

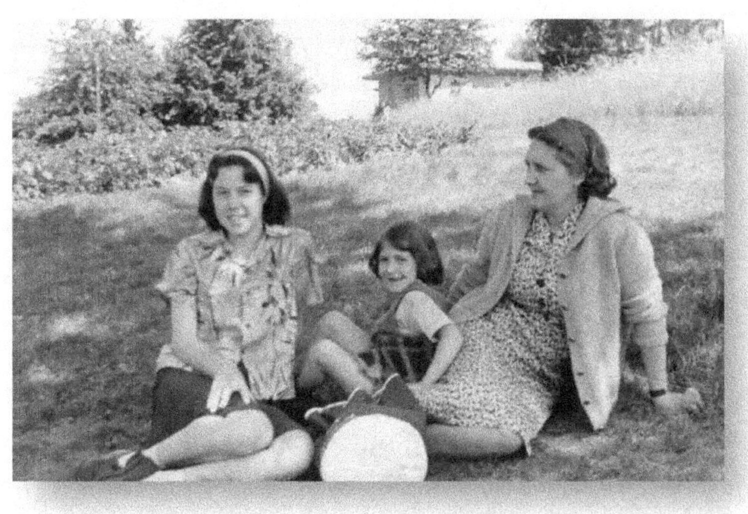

*(Paola with her sister and her mom)*

The first story that comes to mind is my younger sister, Paola.

A few months after my surgery, as I was recovering and going back to my normal life, I heard the alarming news about my younger sister, who lived in BC. The doctors found Paola had an aggressive form of lymphoma, and they had started her treatments.

I was stunned by the news. I had just crossed a dark tunnel myself and was starting to see a looming of light at the end. Now, there was a shadow covering that bright light as I grieved for what my sister had to endure. I knew what she was going through—the disbelief … the fear … the anxiety … the worry … the despair.

When I talked to Paola on the phone, I tried to be cheerful and encouraging, always emphasising hope. However, as the months passed, and she did not get better, as I had, I became quite sad. I could do very little for her, being so far away.

I frequently asked myself, why so bad for my sister, and so much better for me? Why was her cancer so aggressive, while mine had been slow?

The doctors tried several different therapies, and for a while, it looked as if Paola was going into remission. She and her husband came from out west to Ontario to visit our family, and we enjoyed a great time, with shining, renewed hope. We were even planning to celebrate Christmas together at my brother-in-law's family farm. The weeks passed by, and then we learned the disease had reared its ugly head again. The doctors gave Paola more treatments, but this time they didn't work.

Eventually, the disease defeated her. There was no chance of hope, and I heard her cry when she talked to me. It brought such sadness to me that I could not fully enjoy my recovery.

Paola and I had always been very close and invested in each other. My sister was a very talented person. Paola sewed hers and her children's clothing, she could embroider beautiful work, and she took music lessons for voice and piano. It was a wonderful surprise at my wedding when she sang *"The Lord's Prayer"* so beautifully and had all of our guests in tears. So many talents in one person made me miss her more than ever. My family suffered tremendously when Paola announced her diagnosis—an aggressive form of lymphoma. Three years after her diagnosis, she was gone.

The last time I talked to Paola, she confided how she could hardly keep her faith in God. She was in despair, and it broke my heart to hear her talk like that. Our dear mother was with her until the very end, and afterward, she told me, "I wish I had gone instead of my daughter; she was still young with many years ahead." My family and I still grieve the loss of her.

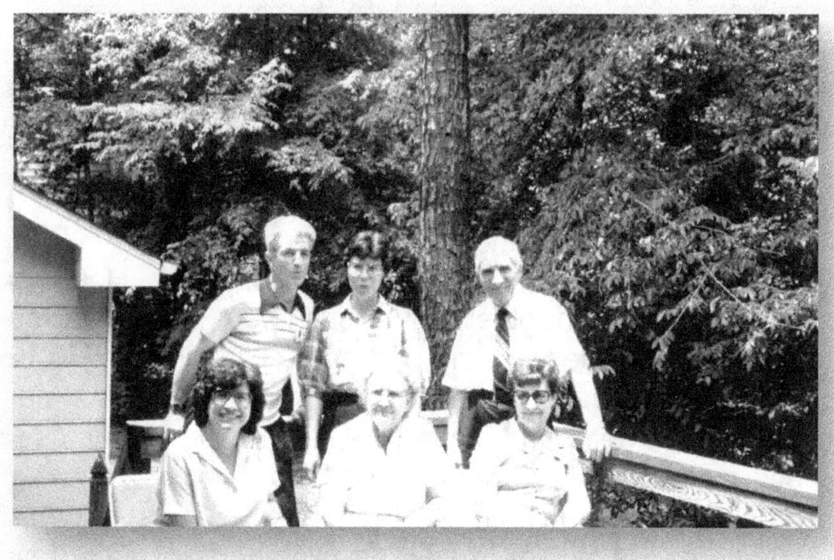

*(Paola with her sisters, brother, & parents)*

# Maggie-Ann's Story

I met Maggie-Ann in Switzerland when I was 22, well before I knew Ernest. We attended the Seminary together, where we studied Theology. It was a painful time in my life, as the young man, whom I thought I loved, suddenly announced his engagement to a woman from his church.

Maggie-Ann didn't know how my feelings were shattered; however, I think she must have sensed something was wrong. She invited me to a share and devotion time before we started our classes and spending time with my new friend seemed to ease my pain. The friendship we formed in Switzerland lasted for years: even after we returned to our home countries, we kept in touch.

Maggie-Ann was from the United States. She and her husband settled in North Carolina, and, coincidentally, she lived only 20 minutes away from my youngest sister. Ernest and I visited Maggie-Ann and her husband, and she and I enjoyed reminiscing about our time in the Seminary. I don't think she ever realized I was in love with that student, but it was not with high regard when she spoke of him.

I was shocked to hear about Maggie-Ann's cancer diagnosis, but her husband told me she fought it courageously. She never allowed cancer to push her down; she continued to travel with her husband, always putting on a cheerful front. She enjoyed my book *"On Call for God,"* and we discussed writing about our time in Switzerland. Maggie-Ann was quite enthusiastic about getting started, but unfortunately, we never got the chance to fulfill that dream.

The last time I visited Maggie-Ann, fear gripped my heart. She didn't look well, although she kept a cheery attitude. I thought this might be the last time I saw her. Ernest took a few photos of all of us, which I cherish. Maggie-Ann had been a happy part of my life and immensely helped me during my time of need. I was not surprised when her husband phoned me with the news of her passing. He told me Maggie-Ann's final months had been agonizing, but she had been courageous to the end.

# Rita's Story

# *One of my neighbours…*

My lovely neighbour, Rita, is well now. I lived beside her at the retirement home. Rita goes out on errands with her family and likes to participate in various retirement home programs.

After her cancer diagnosis, she couldn't accept it because she felt she had lived an everyday, healthy life. Then she had to have heart surgery, which scared her and her family. After Rita recovered from bypass surgery, she had to have blood tests, and that's when the doctors found out she had cancer. Her girls helped her immensely when she started the chemo treatments because they made her quite ill. She told me that she prayed to be taken by God during the nights because she was in so much pain. On top of all this, her husband had died before her diagnosis, and Rita felt very lonely.

Despite her pain, Rita forced herself to get up every day and live her life. She wanted to be strong enough to enjoy her children and grandchildren.

Now she is better and can enjoy many aspects of her life. Rita has accepted that some days are good, and others are not so good, so she takes it easy and enjoys some of the home's activities. She is thankful for every day that she lives. She and I used to go for supper in the main building on Sunday nights, and I look forward to doing that again.

I enjoyed being next door to Rita and chatting with her and watching her beautiful cat when she was away. We went to events together with other friends and genuinely feel that life is good, with many blessings. Even though at the moment, I don't live in the complex, Rita and I still keep in touch.

# Libby's Story

I feel blessed with my close friends throughout the years; they have enriched my life with their attention and wisdom. Libby, a long-time friend, and I enjoy attending church and participating in several events together.

Libby went through cancer, as well. When she discovered she had kidney cancer, she couldn't believe it. The doctors informed her that her cancer was entirely contained; it hadn't spread anywhere. She feels God gave her a miracle because, from the beginning, she felt led by God in doing what she did—being active in the church and helping other people, despite her advanced years.

Our minister gathered a group of Libby's closest friends to pray for her, and then he anointed her. Libby sat in the middle of our group, and each one of us prayed for her.

Before her cancer diagnosis, Libby was thinking about moving to Halifax to be with her son. She was surprised at the results of her ultrasound because she felt no pain. Usually, she felt tired, so she went for a check-up, and the doctor said they had discovered cancer.

Libby had surgery to remove the cancerous kidney, and she stayed in the hospital for four days. When she came home, two ladies from our church looked after her. Libby felt blessed by their care and friendship. Her daughter and grandchildren came from Peterborough to be with Libby, and she was delighted by their presence.

Libby is thankful every day for how she feels now and says she owes it all to God, whom she thanks every day for taking care of her walk with cancer. I am thankful she came into my life many years ago when I moved to this town.

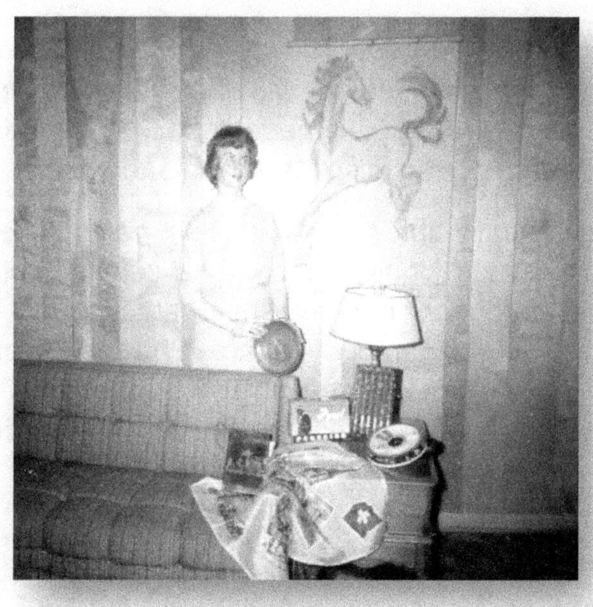

*(Libby)*

# Jeannie's Story

# *Love, laughter, and a healing journey*

*(Note: Jeannie is telling her story, as per her request)*

One of the most dreaded sentences a patient can hear is, "you have cancer." Although there is significant progress in treating this disease, recovery can be long and painful. Cancer is a debilitating and sometimes terminal disease of the body. If an incurable disease has invaded your life, refuse to let it touch your spirit. Your body might be severely afflicted, and you may have a great struggle, but if you keep trusting God's love, your spirit will remain strong——no matter the outcome.

*Psalm 46:1 "God is our refuge and strength, a very present help in times of trouble."*

My trials began in November of 1993. The doctor was crying as she handed me the radiologist's report. Upon reading the ultrasound results, I asked, "You mean, I have cancer?" My abdomen's mass measured about two to three inches high and eight to nine inches long, and a biopsy confirmed Non-Hodgkin's lymphoma. Lymphoma is a blood cancer that affects over 6,000 people each year in Canada. After months of testing and without treatment, I experienced spontaneous remission. My oncologist called me "the mystery lady," but I considered myself "the miracle lady."

Ten years later, in February 2004, I was admitted to the hospital for a hysterectomy. Still, because of my history, my gynaecologist did a laparoscopy first and discovered I had Non-Hodgkin's lymphoma.

The doctor told me that I had a very aggressive form of cancer and would treat it aggressively. So began six months of chemo treatments, CT scans, blood tests, doctor's visits, needles in my stomach to boost my white blood cell count, and even a five day stay in the hospital due to infections. Every three weeks, I had my chemo treatment, which was always preceded by blood work. The human body is an amazing instrument, and it's incredible what we can sustain. We cannot escape pain in this life, but our choice is how we react to it.

Your body has all of these chemicals going into it, and you begin to wonder—what is worse, the disease or the treatment. Taking control of your health becomes your primary focus. The doctors and the drugs were a vital and integral part of my healing. It was essential that I also did my part—I consumed Gatorade by the gallons, I drank Carnation Instant Breakfast, and made homemade milkshakes to build me up.

The less we are in control, the more anxious and worried we become. Being a very independent person—one who is always looking after everyone else—it was challenging to become disabled.

# *Laughter*

Humour is a presence in the world—like grace—and it shines on everybody. I have always loved to laugh, and humour was another sidekick that aided me through my illness. Laughing also helped to ease the pain of those around me. *He who laughs lasts.* If you can laugh despite the circumstances surrounding you, you will enrich others and yourself. Every time I went to the cancer clinic, I emailed family and friends to update them on my progress and used humour to uplift them.

Books like Barbara Johnson's *Pain is Inevitable, but Misery is Optional, so Stick a Geranium in Your Hat and Be Happy* made me laugh. I did my best to surround myself with uplifting things and stay away from the negative.

Eternity is waiting for all of us, but if we can accept the pain that comes into this life and choose to react positively, we can avoid misery. We always have the option to choose joy.

# *Healing*

*For those who trust in the Lord for help will find their strength renewed. They will rise on wings like eagles, they will run and not be weary, and they will walk and not grow weak… Isaiah 40:31*

I have genuinely come to believe that when we are struck down by adversity, God weeps with us and that because we are so loved, He heals us in ways we can never imagine.

When I was travelling this journey, I kept a journal. My journal was on the computer, but I didn't update every day because there were days when I was just too sick. However, it helped me to have a record of what I was going through. I still have the journal I kept from my first bout of cancer. With the cards I received, I had my daughter put them on a "healing tree" with an angel on top. Because I received so many, there became a need for an additional one, which I put in my den, so they were always there to remind me of others' love and support.

# *Faith*

*I am close to you when you are broken-hearted and crushed in spirit. Cast all of your worries upon Me because I care for you. I, even I, am He who comforts you. I'll exchange your sorrow for comfort and joy… Psalm 34:18*

God can take your trouble and change it into treasure. Your misery can become joy—not just a momentary smile but a deep, new joy. We feel God's presence the most when we walk the valleys and feel His gentle arms around us.

Those of us who have faith know that God is a loving Father. Faced with the challenge of illness, we must ask, "If our Father asks us to walk this path rather than another, what blessing does He want to give us now, but cannot?—until we have walked through this suffering with Jesus. And if it is His will for us to be well, He will ensure that we achieve that goal.

# *Hope*

*Do not be afraid- I will save you. I have called you by name—you are mine. When you pass through deep waters, I will be there with you; your troubles will not overwhelm you. When you pass through fire, you will not be burned; the hard trials that come will not hurt you. You are precious to me, and I love you and give you that honour. Do not be afraid; I am with you... Isaiah 43: 1 - 5*

*"In an Instant"* is a book by Bob Woodruff, an anchorman who suffered severe roadside bomb injuries. His wife, Lee, writes:

*We have to choose to laugh and keep smiling. We have to hope there is always something better around the corner. We have to dig down, believe unfailingly in the human spirit's ability to triumph in ways we didn't think possible. To choose to be resilient, ultimately to bounce back, is to choose to be grateful. I look at the man I chose to walk through this world with, and I feel only love: love and eternal hope.*

*May God, the source of hope, fill you with all joy and peace as you trust in Him so that your hope will continue to grow by the power of the Holy Spirit… Romans 15:13*

# Part Four –

# The Man From Halifax –

# Ernest's Story

As I consider the friends I have included in my book, I would like to mention the man in my life, my husband, who also has been hit by cancer. I am now living apart from Ernest: because of his mental and physical condition, he lives in a long-term care home.

When I visit him in the long term care home, we listen to the music we both enjoy, talk about our past experiences, our children and grandchildren, and our many friends. He still remembers so many people in his life and likes to recall when he lived in Indonesia with his family, where he was born. Therefore, I have included a brief story of his remarkable life, and I have done so with great respect for him.

Ernest has been healthy all his life, hardly suffering a cold. He has always been strong, agile, and fit. I remember him in our garden, playing soccer with our children, running and kicking the ball all the time. Our neighbour, younger than he, watched him with envy.

Ernest's life has been all about caring for his family and friends, so I decided to write about him as the concluding part of my book.

He came from Halifax, where he lived with his family for a long time. His life has been honest, with integrity and hard work. I have always been grateful to the Lord for bringing Ernest into my life and changing it into a serene existence. He changed my life from deep loneliness into a story of calm love and tenderness for him and our family.

When we first met, I was a home missionary, going to people's houses and teaching ESL—English Second Language—in church. However, when I went home after work, I felt so lonely, and this began to weigh heavily on me. My parents and sisters were far away, and even though I had several acquaintances, I didn't feel like I had any real friends. I believe I might even have been depressed before meeting Ernest.

# *Indonesia - Java*

Ernest told me that life was pleasant on the Tea Plantation, near Java, where Ernest's stepfather was the superintendent. There was a variety of many animals and the natives who took care of his family, which included his mother, stepfather, and a baby brother. Ernest's native tongue was Dutch, the family having come from Holland to look for work, and the natives taught the family to speak the country's languages.

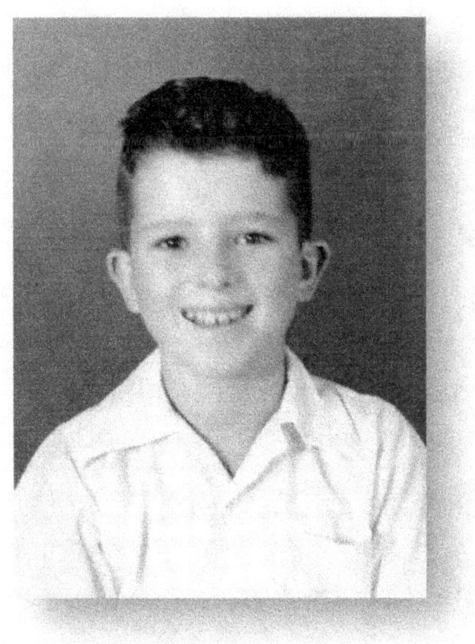

*(Ernest as a boy in Indonesia)*

Ernest's parents listened carefully to the news from Europe and the development of World War II. The announcement was worrisome for them. When the war was declared, the Japanese came to Java and took countless prisoners. Ernest's father was arrested and sent to Burma to work on the famous railroad because he had sabotaged the city's gasoline reservoirs. Ernest, his little brother, and his mother were taken to a concentration camp. His mother was allowed to take only one suitcase and a plate set, and she tied a potty around her waist for Ernest's little brother, Nick. Ernest remembers this well because he was not allowed to take any of his belongings with him. At the time, he did not understand what was happening or why, because he was only three. Ernest learned quickly to obey, stay quiet, and not to speak.

In the camp, life was not pleasant with the Japanese guards and the Commander. The prisoners were not allowed to have a fire, and they were bunked eleven to one room with one window. Food was extremely scarce, most times just a sort of watery porridge and some burnt rice.

Knowing the native languages, Ernest's mother could barter for some food for her and the children, but she had to be careful not to be caught.

At times the Commander would visit the camp, and everyone had to stand at attention and then bow to him. The prisoners had to remain at attention for a long time under the hot sun and listen to the propaganda speeches.

Little Nick died in the camp from whooping cough complications, and Ernest's mother never recovered from his death until the day she died.

Eventually, the war was over, and the prisoners were liberated. After a long trip on a rickety boat, Ernest and his mother reached Holland and lived with Ernest's aunt for a while. Finally, they heard the news that Ernest's stepfather was still alive, and they returned to Java, reuniting the family.

# *Canada*

While in Java, Ernest's **mother** gave birth to two little girls, and eventually, they returned to Holland. However, Ernest's stepfather could not find employment in Holland, so the family immigrated to Canada and settled in Halifax, Nova Scotia.

In the beginning, life was not easy for them, and they all worked hard to make ends meet. Ernest remembers how the entire family went to pick blueberries, which they sold. With that money, he was able to buy a badly needed pair of shoes.

School was not easy, and Ernest was grateful for how everybody helped him to learn English. He excelled, and, still today, his English is excellent. Although life was hard at times, it was much better than in the concentration camp—they were free! The family lived comfortably in Halifax.

After he finished high school, Ernest went to Acadia University to pursue biological studies. He had difficulty with the new math introduced in those years, and in his third year, he left university. Ernest found a job in a photography store, and there he developed his talent for photography, which he used extensively well with his hobby of bird and nature watching. Ernest became a skilful photographer and knew more than 200 different birds just listening to their call, colors, and habits.

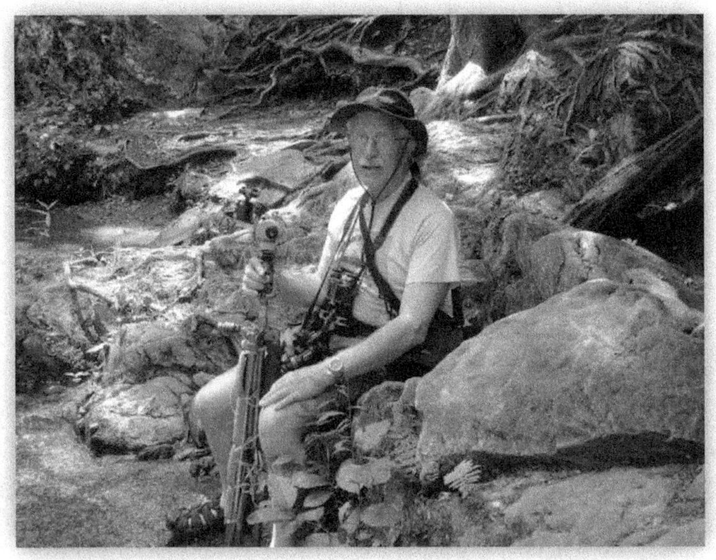

*(Ernest, in North Carolina, bird watching)*

A friend from Montreal called him for the position of Lab Technician in her company, and Ernest moved to Montreal. His life changed. He had his apartment and a beat-up Volkswagen. He attended a nearby Baptist church, as it was his habit of going to church, having found faith in God while frequenting a Halifax youth group.

# A girl in his life

As Ernest attended the church, he became aware of the need for English teachers for the emigrants flooding to Canada in the 1960s. He remembered how people—teachers and students—helped him learn English. Ernest's compassionate heart went out to the hardship numerous emigrants faced in a new country. He decided to help teach English in the teaching centres that were sprouting in Montreal.

The Committee that organized the centres sent him to me, who had just opened a centre in an Italian restaurant in the city's west end. The coordinator of the Centres informed me that a Dutch gentleman from Halifax would come to help me.

Numerous emigrants—Italian, Spanish, and Greek––applied for lessons in my centre, so I was thrilled to receive help in my efforts.

The Dutch gentleman called me, and we settled an appointment at the restaurant to discuss the program. I was excited, especially because his English was flawless with no accent. Although my English had been declared perfect for simple teaching and tutoring, I still had an accent.

I went to the restaurant with expectations. The place was almost empty, except for two men reading newspapers and a young man sitting at a table. Where was my teacher?

I had imagined a middle-aged man, perhaps a family man, but this was not it. He was not there!

Then the young man got up and came to me with a smile and outstretched hand and introduced himself. It was my teacher—it was Ernest—the man from Halifax. I was pleasantly surprised that this distinguished and handsome young gentleman would be my teacher at the centre. We talked for a while and, years later, Ernest told me that he had been so pleased to meet me, such a pretty young lady, who appeared to be bright and in control of her program, so well organized already. He had imagined someone much older.

When we started our classes, the students greeted us with delight and enthusiasm. Ernest took the more advanced levels, where students already had some English knowledge, and I took the beginners. Everybody liked Ernest and took to his friendly, well-trained manners.

After three months, he asked me out, and we started dating. I was thrilled and no longer felt the loneliness that had reigned in my soul for far too long. We had a great year and announced our engagement at Christmas, celebrating a happy time.

# One step to Heaven

After our wedding in Montreal—which was an extremely happy day for our family and us—we became a family and eventually moved to another city with our children. Ernest was an attentive father, not showing much feelings and affection, but caring for his family with hard, steady work. He was a considerate and caring husband to me, always making sure that I was well and had everything I needed. Ernest surprised me sometimes, with little presents, for no particular reason, except that he thought I might like it. He was always ready to take us to appointments or events.

All the homes we had were comfortable, well kept, neat, and lovely. When I had just a few cabinets, Ernest built more for me, painted the rooms, tended the garden, and walked our dog. He volunteered for a time in a prison as a counsellor to prisoners that were halfway ready to re-enter society. He was also active in the church, wherever we were, giving all his support.

In Ernest's spare time, he enjoyed bird watching and taking pictures of nature and wildlife. He became quite skilful in his hobby and in creating a comfortable home for us.

Later on, when I attended university for my Master of Divinity degree, he took me faithfully to the Go-train before going to his work and then would pick me up at the station on my return. When I saw him in our car in the parking lot, I felt safe and well cared for.

Ernest has always been a person who cared for people and animals. His faith in Christ never wavered but encouraged others to believe. One morning, as we were going to the station to catch my train, I complained about how tired I was and how hard life was—caring for the children, for the home, and studying for my degree. It was early in the morning, and the sun was rising. The sky had beautiful flashes of red and golden colors—a stunning display of nature.

Ernest listened to me and then said: "Look at the sky. It tells us God is in control, no matter what." They were simple words but expressed a deep faith, and I kept them precious for the rest of my life. They rendered my husband even more precious to me.

# *Then his health changed.*

After Ernest retired from the firm where he had worked for 27 years, he took other simple jobs until he landed a position as a crossing guard at one of the city schools. He enjoyed this job because he had a chance to talk to the children, learn their names, and get to know their parents. Still today, some of those families remember him. He stayed at this job until he was 74 and then decided it was a bit too much for his age, and he wanted to stay home with me.

While at his different jobs, Ernest also volunteered at the hospital, transporting patients to the Worship Service in the Chapel. He did this for over 20 years, supporting and helping me in my position as Chaplain at the hospital. Together, we helped the hospital and our church as well as we could in our retirement.

We were able to be at home, enjoying a peaceful life in each other's company in our beautiful home and garden. Then I started to notice changes in Ernest, not just aging, but also with his memory. The doctor diagnosed him with mild dementia. Ernest could still drive and have a good conversation, so we took a trip to visit long-time friends. There it happened.

Ernest fell from a long ramp of stairs, losing a lot of blood where his head hit. He was in the hospital for a week before we returned home, with the help of our children.

However, Ernest was not the same. On one of his visits to the doctor, the doctor discovered Ernest had prostate cancer. He also had an MRI on his head, which turned out normal—thank God!

We continued to live at home until I realized its upkeep had become too much for both of us. Ernest could hardly walk and often fell. I was getting overly tired, trying to look after him and the home. We moved to a lovely, comfortable, caring retirement home and enjoyed making new friends, pleasant activities, and a happy, comfortable life together.

Sadly, Ernest's condition took a turn for the worst. He developed urinary infections and had to recuperate in the hospital. Eventually, we admitted Ernest to a Long Term Care facility, where he is now. The difficulty for our family is that Covid 19 developed globally, bringing sacrifices and restrictions. For four months, we were unable to see each other. We had to stay apart for the first time in our married life. It was heart-wrenching.

I kept busy with various pleasurable activities during the day, but at night, I would think so much about him that I cried bitterly and could not fall asleep.

# *What Ernest has given to his family and friends.*

Ernest's life has been a gift of himself to everyone who came into his life. He never showed his feelings openly, but he was always there for his friends in need. He nurtured a constant faith in God by reading his bible and by praying. In this way, he has shown deep care and understanding of people near him. He has not been a *Dad* figure to his children because he never played games with them. But, Ernest was a good *Father* who did everything for his family. He took care if they were sick, helped with school projects, and drove them to places they wanted to go. He has been my faithful companion, supporting and encouraging me in all my endeavours, and I am grateful to him for helping me to develop into what I am today.

He also helped his mother for a long time. She was able to live independently until the end because of her son's assistance and care. Ernest always commented: "She went through a lot for me when I was growing up, now it is my time to look after her." He was with her when she passed away, holding her hand.

When Ernest started to have health problems, he never complained. He always said: "Maybe this is the way my life is going to be from now on. I take what's coming daily." And when he entered the Long Term Care Centre, he said: "I think this is going to be my home now."

I love him with the deep feeling that we have always been good, faithful, and understanding partners for as long as we shall live. We pronounced our vows fifty years ago, "In sickness and in health … for better for worse … till death do us part."

I believe, even then, we will be together with the Lord that we both love and serve.

*(Pictures of me and Ernest throughout our years together)*

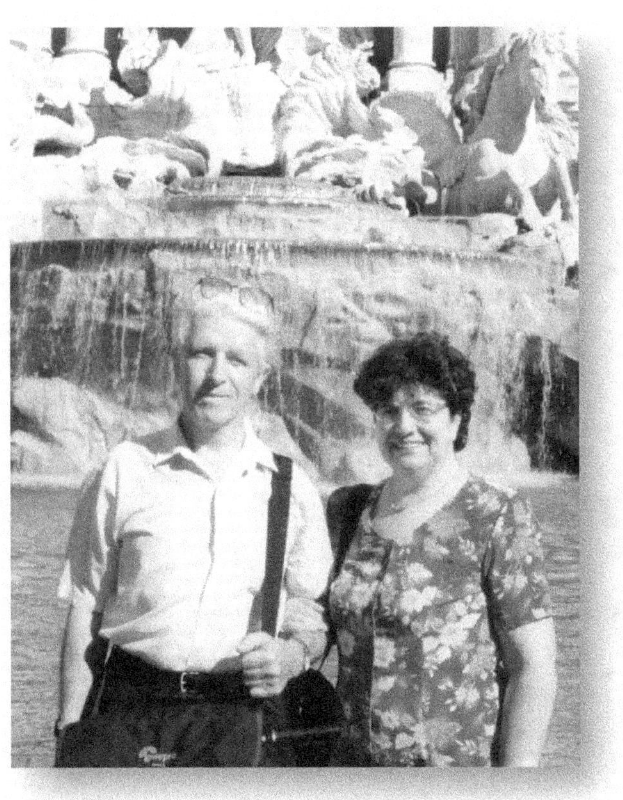

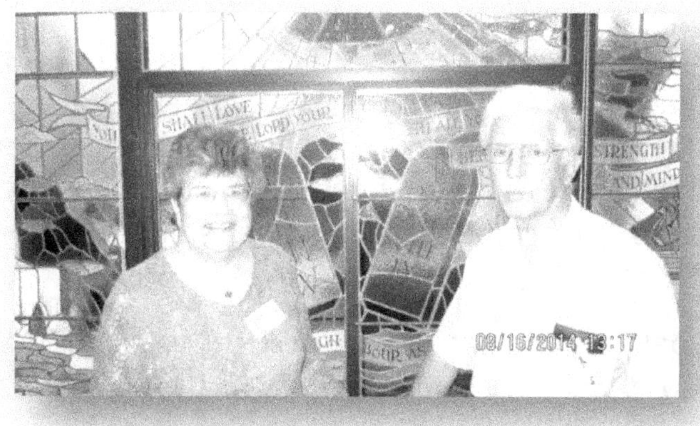

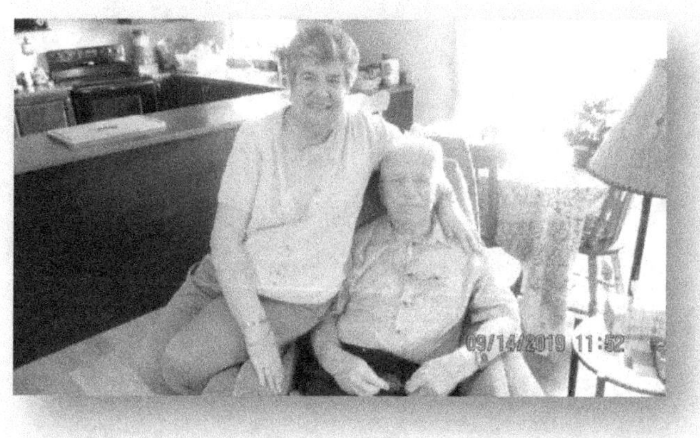

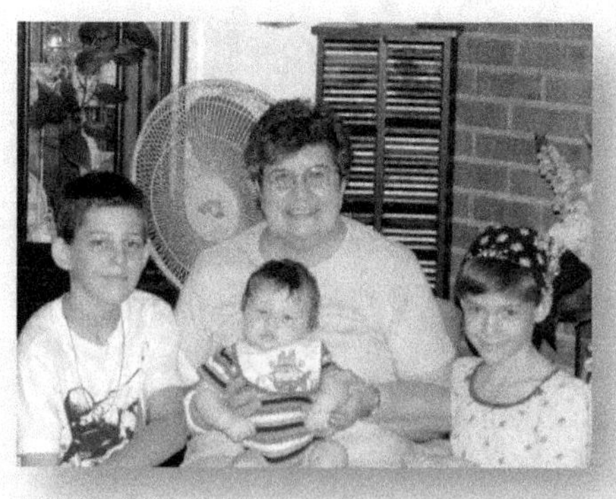

*(My Grandchildren)*

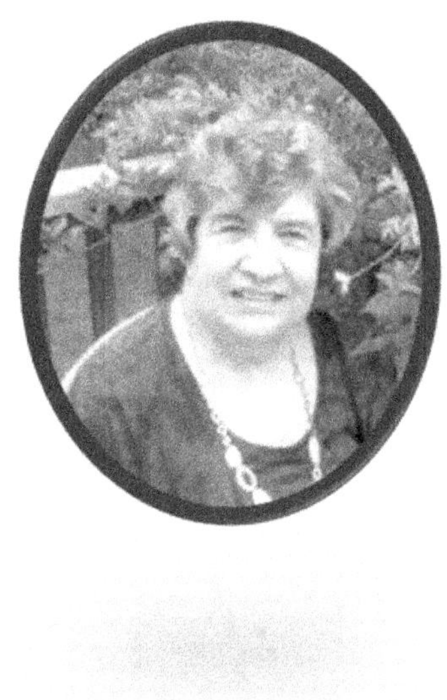

## Mirella Coacci van der Zyl

Mirella Coacci van der Zyl was born in Torino, Italy, during WWII. She was the second of five children of a Baptist minister in Italy. She came to Canada in 1965 and followed theological studies. Eventually, Mirella was ordained into the ministry with the Canadian Baptists of Ontario and Quebec.

After almost twenty years as a chaplain in various hospitals, Mirella retired in 2005 and began her writing career. Her stories have appeared in the local newspaper, *The Brantford Expositor*, and numerous religious magazines. She is the author of *On Call for God*, a book about her experiences as a chaplain; *I Heard the Rumbling of the Planes, Childhood Memories of War*, *Silva's Journey*, *Nonna's Chair*, and *Bullied*.

Mirella now lives in Mt. Pleasant, Ontario, Canada.

# Acknowledgements

This book was in my heart for many years, and I finally found the courage to share it to the public.

Several people helped me to bring to light what was in my heart.

First of all, to my granddaughter, Grace, who typed and corrected my manuscript. I am immensely thankful to her.

To my friends around me, who supported me in this work and contributed to it—I will not name them, but they know I have listened to them and wrote their stories. I sincerely thank them for putting up with me.

Finally, I thank my editor, Mary M. Cushnie-Mansour, and Regina Jetleb, her assistant, for helping me to bring my book to reality. I hope these stories will touch some lives with hope for a better future, not only in this world but in Heaven, as well.

# Cancer Facts & Resources

## Canadian Cancer Society

https://www.cancer.ca

## American Cancer Society

https://www.cancer.org/

According to the highlights from the 2019 publication—Canadian Cancer Statistics—Cancer remains the leading cause of death in Canada. Nearly one in two Canadians will develop cancer in their lifetime, and about one in four will die from cancer. In 2019, an estimated 220,400 Canadians will be diagnosed with cancer, and 82,100 will die from cancer.

The number of cancer cases and deaths remains high in Canada, and, owing to the growing and aging population, it is expected to continue to increase. Although there is progress in reducing deaths for most major cancers (breast, prostate, and lung), there has been limited progress for pancreatic cancer, which the medical community expects to be the third leading cause of cancer death in Canada in 2020. Additional efforts to improve uptake of existing programs and advance research, prevention, screening and treatment are needed to address the cancer burden in Canada.

Cancer poses a large and growing impact on the Canadian population and the health care system. Nearly half of Canadians can expect to receive a diagnosis of cancer in their lifetime. Although age-standardized cancer mortality rates have decreased substantially since they peaked in 1988, cancer remains the leading cause of death among Canadians. Also, the number of new cancer cases and cancer deaths has been increasing each year as the population grows and ages.

Cancer is costly; cancer care costs in Canada rose from 2.9 billion in 2005 to 7.5 billion in 2012. Given the increasing number of cancer diagnoses, the expenses to people with cancer, their families, and the health care system overall are likely to continue to rise in the future.

## Various Questions People Ask About Cancer:

### What are the odds of getting cancer in Canada?

Based on 2015 estimates: Nearly one in two Canadians (45% of men and 43% of women) are expected to develop cancer during their lifetime. About one out of four Canadians (26% of men and 23% of women) are expected to die from cancer.

### What is the leading cause of cancer in Canada?

### Risk Factors

Tobacco use is the cause of almost 30 percent of all fatal cancers in Canada and a major cause of lung cancer, one of the most preventable cancers. Poor Diet—one with a high proportion of dietary fat—causes about 20 percent of fatal cancers.

### Why is cancer so common nowadays?

The main reason cancer risk overall is rising is because of our increasing lifespan. Researchers behind these new statistics reckon that about two-thirds of the increase is due to the fact we're living longer. The rest, they think, is caused by changes in cancer rates across different age groups.

## What percentage of chemo patients survive?

Five years after treatment, 47% of those who got chemo were still alive. The five-year survival rate was 39% among those who did not undergo chemo.

www.ingramcontent.com/pod-product-compliance
Lightning Source LLC
Chambersburg PA
CBHW052203150726
48002CB00003B/1103